Angelic-Reiki Energy Healing Level 2

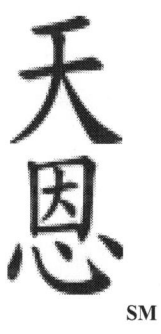

SM

Written By
Rev. Debbie Michaels

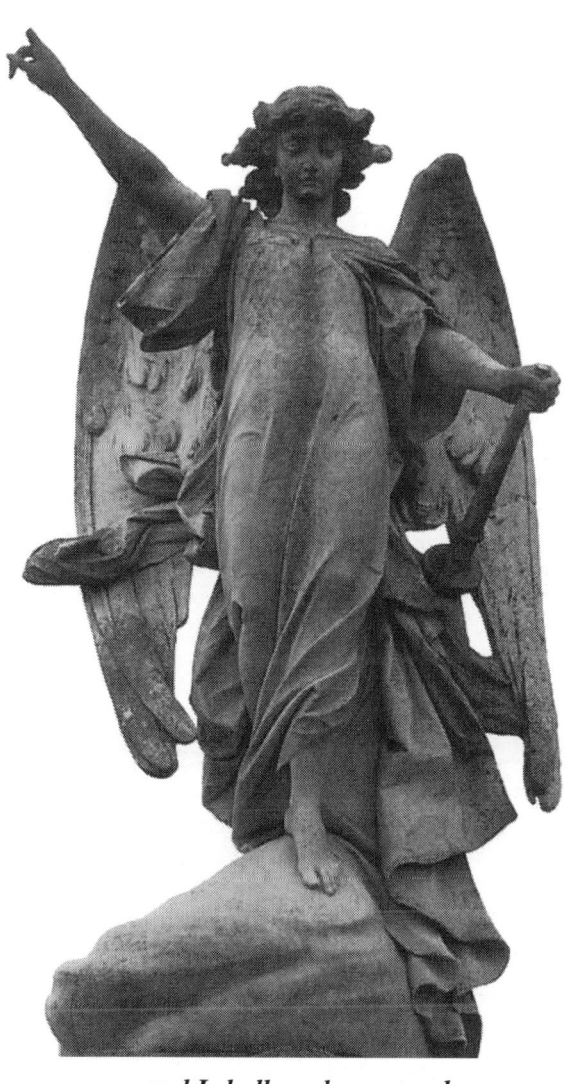

. . . and I shall send you angels
to guard you, to guide you,
and to bless you
Indeed

Attention Future

Angelic-Reiki Energy Healers

All though the Art of *Angelic-Reiki Energy Healing™* is a taught Art, the *Angelic-Reiki Healing Energy* cannot be taught.

Angelic-Reiki Healing Energy is a Gift transferred from Rev. Debbie Michaels God's conduit for *Angelic-Reiki Healing Energy*, to the *Newly Ordained Angelic-Reiki Energy Healing Master*.

The *Angelic-Reiki Energy Healing Program;* is a combination of *Angelic-Reiki Attunements* and *a Gift of Angelic-Reiki Healing Energy*; given through *The Most Sacred Blessing preform by Rev. Debbie Michaels.*

This Blessing May Be Given by Rev. Debbie Michaels, in person or through Distance Blessing. *However, no other Human Being is a Conduit for Angelic-Reiki Healing Energy.*

Angelic-Reiki Energy Healing™ works in harmony with the Human Realm of *Traditional Medicine*.

Angelic-Reiki Energy Healing™ **is not a substitute for Traditional Medicine, but an addition to it.**

We Are Not Medical Doctors.

We Recommend that All Clients Seek Traditional Medical Help by a License Medical Doctor, or Other Health Care Professional; and then abide to their Medical Professional Advise.

By the Grace of God,
Go I

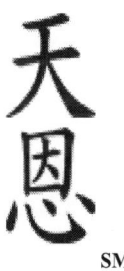

SM

The top symbol represents

GOD

Our Divine Creator

The other symbol represents

GRACE

May the Grace of God find favor in you.

Angelic-Reiki Energy Healing™
Level 2
Written By
Rev. Debbie Michaels

<u>ACKNOWLEDGEMENTS</u>

This book, as all my books are dedicated to
My Guards and My Guides
The Powers That Be
With My Gratitude
Be Blessed
Indeed

Angelic-Reiki Energy Healing™
Level 2
Written By
Rev. Debbie Michaels
Subject to copyright ©

Contact the author at…
www.WhereAngelsGather.org

Angelic-Reiki Energy Healing™
Level 2
Copyright © 2011
Library of Congress Catalog Card Number TX 7-449-388
ISBN 978-1466230880
Where Angels Gather, The Fellowship Inc.
The Fellowship Inc.
Written By
Rev. Debbie Michaels

Contact the author at…
www.WhereAngelsGather.org

About the Author

After a **Death Experience** on January 2, 2003, Debbie Michaels began to hear the Angels speak.

Her Death Experience sent her into a Spiritual Emergence which turned into **a SPIRITUAL EMERGENCY**. She was not aware that this terrifying experience was the beginning of her **Most Sacred Journey**.

To say the least it has changed her life entirely.. She became an Ordained Minister on November 11, 2007 and is the founder of...

> **...Where Angels Gather, The Fellowship Inc.**

Along with her *Death Experience* came many spiritual gifts. Debbie Michaels is a Recognized Clairvoyant, Medical Intuitive, Extreme Empath, Spiritual Healer, Angelic-Reiki Master and Mystic.

She has also been given *The Gift of Being*, and has channeled the following books, in addition to the one you are about to experience.

Angelic Signs and Symbols
The Language of the Angels

Angelic-Reiki Energy Healing
Level 1

The Art of Angelic Ritual Prayer
Manifesting Miracles

The Art of Angelic Ritual Prayer
Handbook of Divine Energy

The Art of Angelic Ritual Prayer
Book of Divine Herbal Energy

Once More

~ Welcome to the Realm of the Angels ~

Table of Contents

Chapter 7
Things to Remember: Angelic-Reiki Procedures

Chapter 8

My Wish for You

Chapter 1

Introduction
Angelic-Reiki Healing Energy
Level 2

Angelic-Reiki Energy Healing Level 2

Introduction:

In Level 2 the Practitioner will learn the Angelic-Reiki Symbols and the purpose for using these Sacred Symbols. The practitioner will also learn the correct hand placement to permit the very best energy flow.

In addition the practitioner will learn the different Angelic-Reiki Healing Techniques, that they will have available to offer their clients.

The Practitioner will also learn to work with their clients Traditional Medical needs; honoring the Human anatomy and the requirements of their Earthly Human Body.

Angelic-Reiki Energy Healing™ Level 2 includes the practitioner's second attunement, and just as with, your *first attunement* in Level 1, there will be another 40 day adjustment period. During this period, you, the future *Angelic-Reiki Energy Healer™*, will experience many more Spiritual Gifts. Your personal attunement will open you up more spiritually than you have ever been before.

The practitioner will be able to sense energy more easily, and will also become more telepathic and clairvoyant (the practitioner will begin to see energy and how it flows). And that will be only the beginning; the spiritual gifts that you already have will become amplified. But not to worry along with the amplification will come the capability to handle these gifts. *They will become only gifts, not burdens.*

Angelic-Reiki Energy Healing™
Level 2…

…is a gift that is now being given to you, the practitioner; use it Knowingly for with this Knowledge you will bring healing, use it with Love for with Love you will show Compassion, use it within the Light for Angelic-Reiki Energy Healing™ comes from The Light of The Angelic-Reiki Realm; The Realm of The Divine Healing Angels.

Chapter 2

Angelic-Reiki Energy Healing Empowerment Attunement

Angelic-Reiki Energy Healing Empowerment Attunement

This *Second Angelic-Reiki Energy Healing Attunement* connects the practitioner to the Angelic-Reiki Realm of Energy Healing Angels; and the Angelic-Reiki Healing Energy; which you will continue to channel as you open up to your Divine mission as an *Ordained Angelic-Reiki Energy Healing Master.*

The Practitioner will use their *Gift* to help facilitate the healing process of the Human Being. This healing energy may be used both on one's self and also on the Clients you will *service.*

For as an Angelic-Reiki Energy Healer, the practitioner will be of service to the Human Being.

The *Second Angelic-Reiki Attunement* strengthens the practitioner's healing gifts and will *empower* them on many levels. Each level of the *Angelic-Reiki Energy Healing Attunements* process will also strengthen the practitioner's auric field and also the *Angelic Chakra Alignment* that was received during the First *Angelic-Reiki Attunement.*

The *Second Angelic-Reiki Attunement* process itself involves **Rev. Debbie Michaels** connecting with the student on a *Divine Angelic-Reiki Energy Level*; the practitioner is then connected *permanently* to this *Angelic-Reiki Energy Level*.

The *Second Angelic-Reiki Attunement* involves opening up the practitioner's energy channels with distinct focus upon the Crown and Third-Eye chakras. This opening will also empower the practitioner's palms with Angelic-Reiki Healing Energy; which will be used for Spiritual Healings. We heal from the inside, out, we heal all dis-ease (disease) of the Soul, and this healing transforms into the physical healing.

The *Second Angelic-Reiki Energy Healing Attunement* is a process of empowerment that opens the crown, heart and palms of the practitioner connecting their body to the **Unlimited Source** of *Angelic-Reiki Healing Energy*. During and after this *Sacred Second Angelic-Reiki Attunement* subtle changes are brought about to cleanse and heal the practitioner in order to become a more effectively Spiritual Healer. **Note:** These changes take place on all levels, physical, mental, emotional and spiritual, this adjustment period, as with the first Angelic-Reiki Attunement will last another 40 days.

Preparing for the Level 2 Angelic-Reiki Energy Healing Attunement

In order to improve the results of your receiving of the *Angelic-Reiki Energy Healing Second Attunements*, a process of purification is recommended. This will allow the attunement energies to work more efficiently and create better benefits for you. *The following steps are simply suggestions, follow them if you feel guided to do so:*

- Increase water intake for three days.

- Avoid alcohol for at least three days prior to the attunement.

- Avoid foods with artificial additives.

- Meditate each day for a half hour; using any form you are accustomed to.

- Spend some time in silence each day for a week prior to the attunement.

Following these guidelines is an individual decision, but I do emphasize that a few days of purification will enhance the wonderful and powerful experience of the *Angelic-Reiki Energy Healing Second Attunement.*

An ***Angelic-Reiki Energy Healing Attunement*** is an acknowledgment of the practitioner's connection and commitment to Angelic Healings. By receiving this attunement the practitioner will become part of an elite group of people who are initiated into ***The Realm of Angelic-Reiki Energy Healing.***

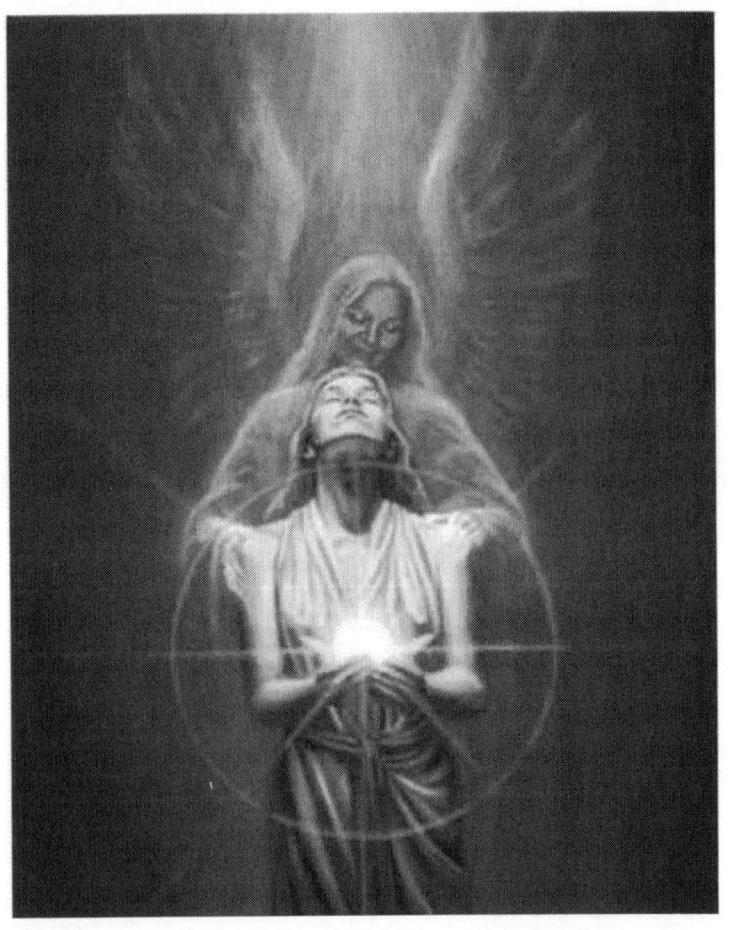

Physical Purification:

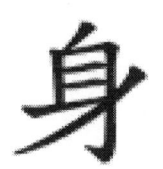 When Angelic-Reiki is purifying the student's physical body, minor flu-like symptoms may be experienced: and minor discomforts include achy muscles, headache, constipation, or diarrhea, and other symptoms. As toxins are being released, odors in the urine and feces may also occur.

To lessen the effects: spend extra time doing *Angelic-Reiki Energy Healing* on one's self, over symptomatic areas; breathe clean fresh air deeply into the lungs, and drink lots of pure fresh water. Eat light nourishing meals which include fresh fruits, vegetables and juices. Also it is very important that you get plenty of rest. A minimum on 8 hours of sleep is recommended for at least one week after the attunement. After that a minimum of 6 hours should be enough, but this requirement will differ with each individual.

Please, it is asked of you to follow the suggestions stated above.

<u>Notes</u>

Emotional Purification:

情 During this purification of the emotional body, deeply held emotions may surface, such as anger, frustration, grief, fear, and sadness. These emotions may have been blocked or repressed from earlier experiences.

These emotions are being released from the depths of the student's physical conditions; from their cellular level of body and mind. Please do not place blame on yourself, anyone, or anything, for these feelings. Just experience them as they surface and let them go. Seek spiritual counselling if necessary.

<u>**To lessen the effects**</u>, place one power-hand on your *Third-Eye Chakra* and the other over your *Sacral Chakra*. Breathe in and visualize *Angelic-Reiki Healing Energy* coming into your crown chakra, circulating throughout your body, and collecting all of the emotional remains; then breathe out forcefully, releasing these negative energies. Keep this up until you feel calm. Take a long hot bath with a teaspoon of **Angelic-Reiki Energy Healing Blessed Salt™;** soak for about twenty minutes. This will relax you and help to cleanse the student's emotional body, be kind to yourself. Repeating positive affirmations and listening to your favorite music will also help ease these negative emotions.

Notes

Mental Purification:

When mental purification is in process, you may notice your thoughts of past events may surface; these thoughts may also be from *Past-Life Events*. Old thought forms, and past behaviour patterns may return. You may become surrounded by thoughts of judgment, blame, victimization, abuse, denial, self-destruction and self-pity. Let those thoughts go and change your thoughts to positive ones; thoughts of moving forward in your life; harmoniously and peacefully.

To lessen the effects, spend extra time doing *Angelic-Reiki Energy Healing* on yourself. This alone can and will move you through the purification process. Talk to like-minded people about your experiences, do things that make you feel happy, build new memories. You may repeat positive affirmations, mantras, and listen to your favorite music. Music has a very healing effect on the mental level.

Notes

Soul Purification:

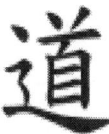 When spiritual purification is in process, your beliefs may be shaken and challenged; beliefs in how the world operates, how relationships should be, and what is important in your life. As this occurs, insights, revelations, and new understanding will become clear; these will be the building blocks of your newly forming and ever-changing soul-foundation.

To lessen the effects, spend extra time doing *Angelic-Reiki Energy Healing* on yourself. Talk to like-minded people about your experiences, read uplifting spiritual books, listen to motivational tapes, and treat yourself with love and kindness. Be open to new thought patterns, for you are evolving.

In Addition:

A person who is called to *Angelic-Reiki Energy Healing*, on all levels of their being, may over a period of time (usually two to three years) experience another purification cycle. This is normal; it is simply keeping the practitioner a pure channel for *Angelic-Reiki Energy Healing*.

<u>Notes</u>

Chapter 3

Traditional
Japanese Reiki

<u>Traditional Japanese Reiki History</u>

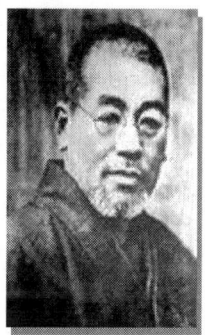

Dr. Usui discovered Reiki during a mystical experience on Mt. Kurama, a Sacred Mountain north of Kyoto, Japan in March of 1922.

He founded the Usui Reiki Healing Society; Dr. Usui began to treat patients shortly after his mystical experience. As the popularity grew for Reiki, Dr. Usui began to train students in this *mystical healing art.*

Reiki teachers and practitioners abide by these five simple teachings.

At least for today:
Do not be angry,
Do not worry,
Be grateful,
Work with diligence,
Be kind to people.

Traditional Japanese Reiki Symbol

Usui Reiki symbols are sacred

The symbols are used to help people focus to connect to Universal Energy. Some people make the error of assuming that the symbols embody the power of Reiki and completely rely on the symbols. *Symbols serve a purpose. They do carry Sacred Energy.* With Traditional Reiki, the Universal Energies are called upon; but these Sacred Symbols are just a part of the process.

Reiki symbols are taught during the Second Degree of Reiki by a Reiki master. In the past, these Reiki symbols were considered sacred. They were used only with the highest integrity. Reiki masters passed these symbols onto their students, but copies were not allowed to leave the teaching areas. Reiki masters helped their students memorize the symbols in the class, this may account for the many variations today; for each person may visualize these symbols differently.

The symbol targets the subconscious mind. The Reiki symbols aren't harmful. It's possible for different Reiki masters to use different Reiki symbols in their teachings with all the variations out there today.

<u>**Traditional Reiki Symbols:**</u>
Please understand it is considered that all writings about Spiritual Matters are Sacred Teachings; and when being shown to an individual a ***Divine Seed*** is planted within the individual; accelerating their spiritual growth and enlightenment.

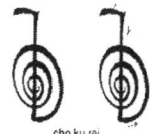

	No. 1.
	Focus. = **Power Symbol** = **Cho ku Rei**

Cho ku rei (cho koo ray) (long o in cho) is the Usui power symbol to increase the power of Reiki . This energy calls in higher universal energy and accelerates Reiki from low to high and gives greater power and focus to the energy .Power boost is used with the other energies as well as by itself during all treatments hands on or distance.

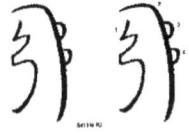

> **No. 2.**
> **Harmony. = Mental**
> **Emotional = Sei he ki**

Sei he ki is the mental emotional healing function Usui mantra is sei he ki (say hay key). The mental emotional function is used to facilitate emotional and mental healing and to assist self-programming and treating addictions and habits as well as all other mental and emotional concerns, it is said to work on the subconscious.

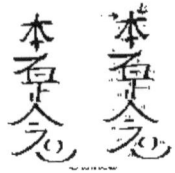

> **No. 3**
> **Connection. = Distance =**
> **Hon sha ze sho nen**

Hon sha ze sho nen is the Distance energy attunement also gives you the ability to use all the Reiki energies for hands off treatments at any distance at all.

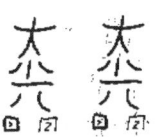

**No. 4
Empowerment. = Master =
Dai ku Myo**

Dai ku Myo is the Third Degree symbol adds the symbol for Self-empowerment, Intuition, Creativity, and Spiritual connection it enables recognition and clarity about your true path.

Notes

Chapter 4

Angelic-Reiki
Energy Healing Symbols

Angelic-Reiki Energy Healing Symbols

During this second level of *Angelic-Reiki Energy Healing* training, the flow of the Angelic-Reiki Healing Energy within you will intensify. You will further enhance your healing abilities through the use of *The Sacred Angelic-Reiki Energy Healing Symbols* bestowed upon you.

Angelic-Reiki Symbols:

Angelic-Reiki Energy Healing like Traditional Reiki makes use of *Sacred Symbols*.

Just as the Second degree of *Angelic-Reiki Energy Healing Attunement* leads the practitioner to the deeper understanding of the Power of the Angelic-Reiki Healing Angels. The use of Their Sacred Angelic-Reiki Energy Healing Symbols will tap into the Divine Healing Power of the Angelic-Reiki Healing Realm.

You will be able to *transcend time and space* with your Angelic-Reiki Energy Healing Abilities.

The Realm of Angelic-Reiki Healing Angels asks that the Human Being always honor all *Sacred Symbols*, for all *Sacred Symbols* come from our **Divine Creator** and carry **Divine Energy**.

Please understand that the receiving of *Angelic-Reiki Energy Healing Symbols* is a part of the Second Sacred Angelic-Reiki Attunement. This attunement will be a change in the practitioner's cellular and genetic levels.   This continues the evolution of the practitioner's mind, emotions, body, and soul.

Angelic-Reiki Energy Healing Practitioners have found that along with the **Angelic-Reiki Energy Healing Attunements,** the use of the **Sacred Angelic-Reiki Energy Healing Symbols** increases their intuitive and psychic awareness. This increase of psychic intuition gives the practitioner the intuitive knowledge of their client's Soul; it's condition and needs.

With this increased knowledge the practitioner is better able to service their client, on all levels, in all realms, and also in all times. Healing not only their present *Soul Dis-ease,* but also any that the client may carry with them form past lives; healing also the Karma which goes with their *Soul Dis-ease*.

The Angelic-Reiki Energy Healing Symbol
"Body" carries the energy of Angelic-Reiki Realm
and Human Being coming together. The primary use
of this Sacred Angelic-Reiki Symbol is to increase
the healing power for the physical body. It draws the
Angelic-Reiki Energies and focuses it to where the
healing is required. It can be used for anything,
anywhere.

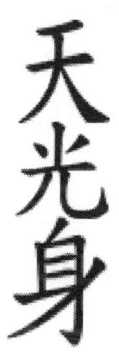

* For on the spot treatments.

* To cleanse negative energies.

* Spiritual protection.

* To aid any physical healing be it
structural or biological.

* In sick rooms and hospitals.

Invoke: Archangel Raphael

Envision this sign over the client
(or yourself) and say (silently)
the words…

*"I ask for Divine Angelic-Reiki Healing Energy to
enter this Physical Body of this Sacred Human
Being, this most Holy Vessel."*

Notes

The Angelic-Reiki Energy Healing Symbol
"Emotion "carries the energy of Divine healing power of Love. It is used primarily for emotional healing. It is the Angelic-Reiki Symbol to use for healing the emotions; it empowers the practitioner with Divine Energy of affection, love, compassion, and sympathy. It is used to heal not only a person's emotions but also for the circumstances that the person may be experiencing.

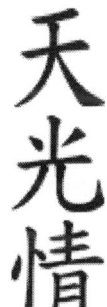

* For on the spot treatments.

* To cleanse negative energies.

* For healing past traumas

* Clears emotional blockages

Invoke: Archangel Muriel

Envision this sign over the client (or yourself) and say (silently) the words…

"As I am one with Angelic-Reiki Healing Energy, I am secure and at peace with myself, I am whole and complete."

Notes

The Angelic-Reiki Symbol "Mind "carries the energy of Divine healing power of Clarity. It is used primarily for mental/emotional healing and calming of the mind. It is used for:

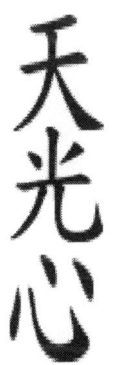

* Psychic protection

* Cleansing

* To balance the right and left brain

* Aid for removing addictions

* For healing past traumas

* Removing negative energies and bad vibrations

Invoke: Archangel Uriel

Envision this sign over the client (or yourself) and say (silently) the words...

"I ask for Clarity, Knowledge, and Wisdom to become one with this Sacred Human Being."

Notes

The **Angelic-Reiki Symbol "Soul"** carries the energy used to heal the soul. Since it deals with the Soul and the Human Being's Spiritual Self, it heals dis-ease and illness from the original source. It helps to provide enlightenment and peace. With the use of this Sacred Symbol the Human Being becomes more intuitive and psychic.

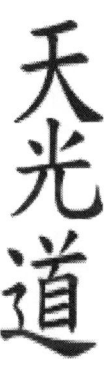

- With repeated use of this most Sacred Symbol you will experience profound life changes

- Heals the Sacred Human Soul

- Balances the Standard Chakras

- Removes negative energy from all layers of the Aura

Invoke: **Archangel Metatron**

Envision this sign over the client (or yourself) and say (silently) the words...

"I accept this Angelic-Reiki Energy Healing. As I am one with The Angelic-Reiki Energy, it Flows freely and in Abundance; Healing the Soul of this your Most Sacred Human Being."

Notes

Learn these Sacred Angelic-Reiki Energy Healing Symbols, for they carry Divine Angelic-Reiki Healing Energy.

These Sacred Symbols may be drawn over the client, or visualizes them during their treatment. You may also choose to place the *Angelic-Reiki Symbol Cards*™ in plain view while you are doing a healing session; this will help the practitioner focus.

Another option is for the practitioner to have their client hold a card with the *Angelic-Reiki Energy Healing Symbol* pictured on them; this method is extremely powerful for both the practitioner and their client.

Notes

Infusing the Student with Energy of the Symbols:

Angelic-Reiki Energy Healing Symbols are the Sacred Symbols used to enhance the flow of the practitioner's healing energy. They are the keys to higher awareness levels and manifestations. These Angelic-Reiki symbols are used by *Ordained Angelic-Reiki Masters* to provide their students and clients with a way to link the image to the Sacred Angelic-Reiki Healing Energies represented in the Angelic-Reiki Symbols.

The *Angelic-Reiki Energy Healing Symbols* are keys that open the doors to miracles, it is necessary for the practitioner to look at these symbols as elements that assist you in the channeling of *Angelic-Reiki Healing Energy* in a precise form. This means that the symbols do not create healings by themselves but act as aids in the process.

Please learn these Most Sacred Angelic-Reiki Healing Symbols, They Carry Divine Healing Energy.

Note: The practitioner is infused with the Energies of these Sacred Symbols during the Second Attunement given by Rev. Debbie Michaels.

Notes

The Fifth Symbol (The Master Symbol)

The Fifth Most Sacred of All Angelic-Reiki Symbol is the *Ordained Master Symbol*. This Most Sacred Symbol is the *central essence of Angelic-Reiki Energy Healing. The Fifth Scared Ordained Master Symbol carries the Angelic-Reiki Light of the Ordained Master.*

This Sacred Symbol is given at the Final Attunement; this is part of a Divine Blessing and the Infusion of Angelic-Reiki Healing Energy. *It signifies the Activation of Angelic-Reiki Healing Energy into the Practitioner.*

This Most Sacred of All Symbols will not be found in this book or any other book. It is kept *Sanctified* by the *Ordained Angelic-Reiki Master*; it becomes a part of their Sacred Being, their Sacred Soul. *This Symbol is not to be shown to anyone.*

The Fifth Angelic-Reiki Master Symbol is given to the newly Ordained Angelic-Reiki Master by Rev. Debbie Michaels during the final attunement at the practitioner's ordination.

This Sacred Angelic-Reiki Energy Healing Ordination may be performed as a Distance Ordination or in person.

Notes

Chapter 5

Anatomy Healing Guide

Divine Life Energy Flow:

All substance, living and non-living, is composed of, and infused with this Divine Energy.

Just as we need blood to flow freely through our body, we also need The Divine Energy to flow freely.

There is within all things an energy system similar to the Human Being circulatory system; it is referred to as the Meridians. Essentially you may say that the Meridians are the equivalent of our blood vessels but instead of transporting blood this system transports our Divine Life Energy.

Dis-ease can occur when there is a blockage in the meridians and the energy no longer can flow freely or when the Meridians are out of balance.

There are two systems of networks within the meridians, that is to say, there are primary and secondary meridians. Primary meridians pass through internal organs however, secondary do not. There are 12 pairs of primary meridians with energy flowing in continuous circulation through the following organs: lungs, colon, stomach, spleen, heart, intestines, urinary bladder, kidneys, gall bladder and liver.

The primary meridians are named by the organ they are connected to i.e. lung meridian, heart meridian etc.

It is important to understand though the meridians are named according to the organs they pass through, this does not mean that they only correspond to those organs. The meridians also consist of complex unified systems for the circulation of the Divine Energy of Life.

The Divine Life Energy contains two polar forces, the *Heavens' Energy* and the *Earth's Energy*. When both are balanced, the Human Being exhibits good physical health; when they are unbalanced, a diseased condition will begin to develop.

Angelic-Reiki treatment will balance the Meridians and enable a smooth flow of Divine Life Energy through the meridian system. Blockages in meridians can be dissolved by Angelic-Reiki Energy Healing and help restore the body's healthy flow of energy.

The 12 Meridians

The Heart Meridian

The Heart Meridian, this meridian represents compassion and thus governs emotions and the soul. It is also responsible for the circulation of the blood through the total body including the brain and the five senses. .

The Liver Meridian

The Liver Meridian, this meridian stores nutrients and energy for physical body. It also helps resists against dis-ease and supplies, evaluates and detoxifies blood in order to maintain good physical health and energy.

The Intestine Meridian

The Intestine Meridian, this meridian helps the function of the lung, from inside and outside the body. It also eliminates any stagnation of energy.

The Triple Warmer Meridian

The Triple Warmer Meridian, this meridian is different from the other meridians because it is not represented by any physical organ. Its purpose is to circulate energy throughout the organs.

The Urinary Bladder Meridian

The Urinary Bladder Meridian is related to the brain, kidney system, and the pituitary gland. It is also connected to the autonomic nervous system related to the reproductive and urinary organs.

The Gall Bladder Meridian

The Gall Bladder Meridian dispenses nutrients through the body and balances the energy with the help of internal hormones and secretions include bile, saliva, gastric acid, insulin, and intestinal hormones.

The Lung Meridian

The Lung Meridian is the intake of Heavenly Energy from the air for use by the body, and to build up resistance against any external disturbances. It also removes gasses that are not required in the body through exhalation.

The Colon Meridian

The Colon Meridian helps the total body through the movement and digestion of food. Anxiety, anger, nervous shock, and emotional excitement can affect the circulation of the blood, and the small intestine can actually cause blood stagnation and may affects the body as a whole.

The Stomach Meridian

The Stomach Meridian is intricate in the workings of the stomach, esophagus, and duodenum, as well as the functioning of the reproductive, lactation, ovary, and appetite mechanism.

The Spleen Meridian

The Spleen Meridian involves the digestion. The spleen governs general digestion, and reproductive hormones related to the breasts and ovaries. Mental fatigue has a negative effect on the spleen and a lack of exercise will cause problems with digestion and also with the secretion of hormones.

The Pericardium Meridian

The Pericardium Meridian acts as a additional function of the heart and circulatory system, which includes the heart sac, the cardiac arteries and the system of arteries and veins. It is also responsible for over-all nutrition.

The Kidney Meridian

The Kidney Meridian, this meridian controls the essence and energy to the body and governs fighting against mental stress by controlling hormone secretions. It also purifies the blood.

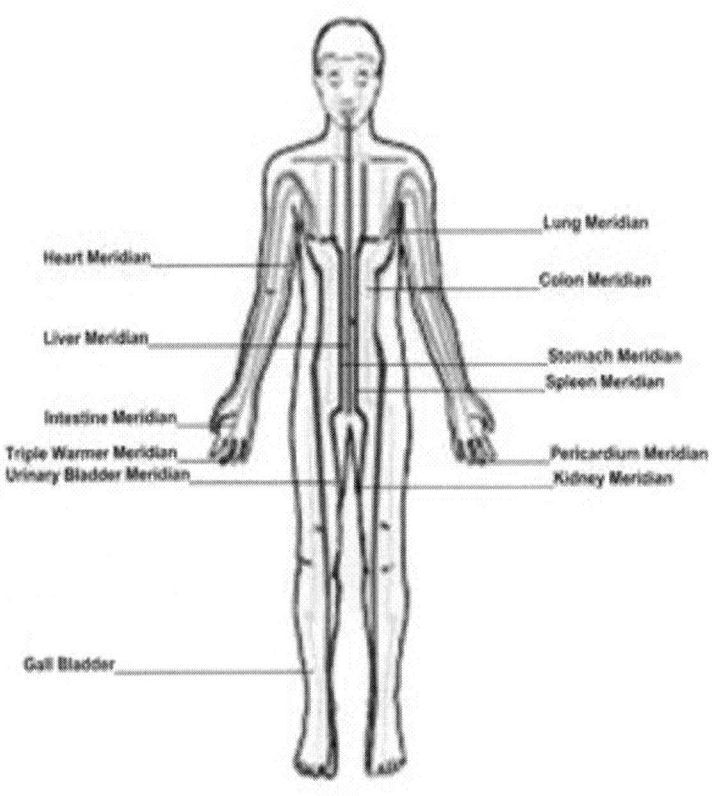

Directing the Flow of Angelic-Reiki Energy:

- Ask your client to lie down on the massage table.

- The room should be dimly lit and comfortably warm so the patient is comfortable.

- Place your hands above the client in the Angelic-Reiki (triangular hand position.)

- Begin by balancing your client's Standard Chakra System.

- Have your client turn over and repeat the positions over the same chakras.

- Wait at each chakra for several minutes. Until you feel the throbbing in your hands.

- Feel the energy from the Angelic-Reiki Angels enter your body and flow through your hands to your client.

- Let your client know to expect a warm feeling of energy (Explain to the client that this is the Angelic-Reiki Healing Energy that they are experiencing.)

- By moving your hand over each chakra, you begin to direct the Angelic-Reiki Healing Energy.

- This is beginning of directing and activating the Angelic-Reiki Healing Energy to flow to where the client needs balance and healing.

Angelic-Reiki Energy Healing Treatment

The effectiveness and ease of use in the Angelic-Reiki Energy Healing system is based on the hand positions of Traditional Reiki. The Angelic-Reiki hand positions are similar to Traditional Reiki, as we are working within the same parameters, (the Human Body).

The Angelic-Reiki Energy Healing hand positions cover all the chakras and also the meridians.

Angelic-Reiki Energy Healing is usually given as a whole body healing treatment, however at the Client's request you may be asked to only focus on one area. *The Angelic-Reiki Practitioner should always honor the request of their client.*

Other times the Angelic-Reiki Practitioner will need to listen to their intuition and receive the guidance from the Angelic-Reiki Realm of Angels, as to the requirements for the clients healing. This is one reason why the practitioner psychic gifts will be intensified.

A full treatment will take just over an hour. A full Session may also include a Standard Chakra Balancing, Soul Event Cord Release (if necessary) and/or an Aura Clearing.

Notes

Notes

Notes

Angelic-Reiki Hand Positions and Procedures:

During an Angelic- Reiki treatment, the hand positions are given with the hands approximately 2 inches from the client's body. The hands should be slightly cupped, the fingers together.

There are twelve Angelic-Reiki hand positions.

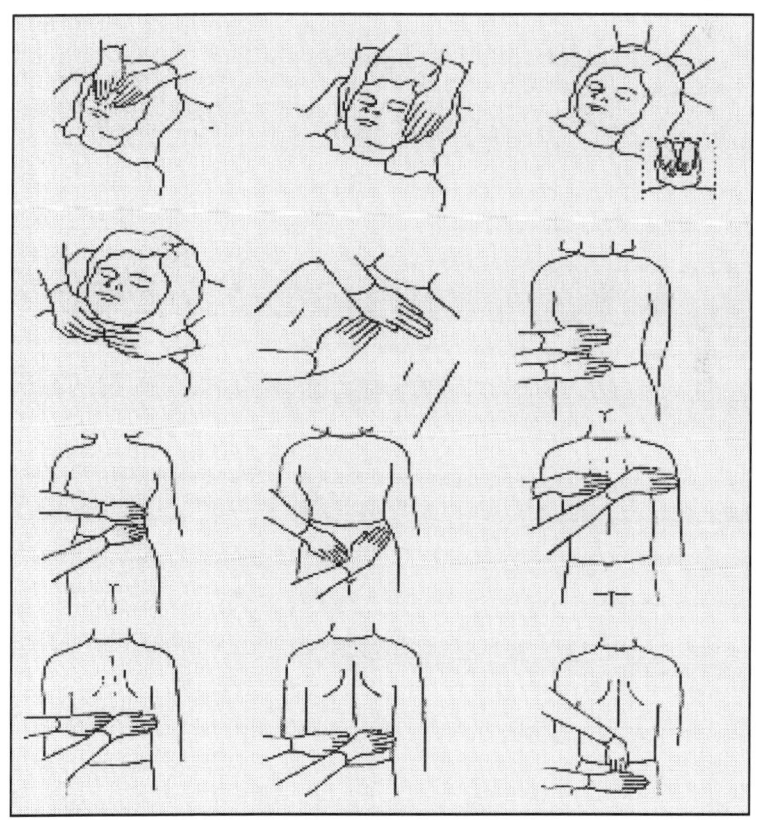

Notes

Position 1:

Angelic-Reiki Energy Healing First Step:

Begin by spraying three sprites of Angelic-Reiki Energy Healing Charge Holy Water™; one spray over the crown chakra, the second over the trunk of the client, and the third at the feet of the client. This prepares the client to receive Angelic-Reiki Healing Energy.

The practitioner's hands are placed over the client's face, palms over the forehead, fingers cupped lightly over the eyes. Be sure to keep the nostrils open at all times.

You will begin to feel the Angelic-Reiki Healing Energy pulse through your hands, once the throbbing begins hold that position, until the throbbing begins to ease up.

Once the pulsing has eased up, lift your hands up above the clients face.

Angelic-Reiki Energy Healing Second step:

You begin by sweeping the client's negative energy that you have pulled out of them, down and away from the client's body.

This is done by a gentle sweeping effect with hands over the face.

> **Note: After completing each treatment position, the Angelic-Reiki practitioner will sweep the client's Aura to clear away the debris that have been lifted during the treatment.**

Once you have completed sweeping the clients facial area, it is now time for the third step.

Angelic-Reiki Energy Healing Third step:

The practitioner will return their hand back to the facial area of the client, but this time the Angelic-Reiki practitioner will have their hands in the (triangular position). You will hold this position until you begin to feel the warmth of the Angelic-Reiki Healing Energy flow through you and into your client.

What is happening at this point is the Angelic-Reiki Angels through the practitioner are infusing Angelic-Reiki Healing Energy into the client; sealing any and all energy holes.

These energy holes must be filled and sealed immediately to prevent any negative energy from gathering again.

Position 2: wrap your hands around the client's head, with your fingertips touching their ears.

Once again you will begin to feel the Angelic-Reiki Healing Energy pulsating through your hands.

Hold that position, until the throbbing begins to ease up.

Once the pulsing has eased up, remove your hands from this position.

Begin the *second* Angelic-Reiki Energy Healing step, by sweeping the client's negative energy that you have pulled out of them, down and away from the client's body.

Once you have completed the sweeping, it is now time to perform the *third* step.

The practitioner will return their hand back to the ear area of the client, and place their hands in the (triangular position). The Practitioner will hold their hands over their client's ear, starting with the right ear and then moving to the left ear. You will hold this position over each ear until you begin to feel the warmth of the Angelic-Reiki Healing Energy flow through your hands and into your client.

> **Repeat all three Angelic-Reiki Steps with each additional position.**

Position 3:

Tuck your hands gently underneath the client's head, forming a cradle.

Position 4: Surround your client's jaw line with your hands allowing your fingertips to touch underneath the client's chin.

Position 5: Place your left hand over the heart center while your right hand is lightly hovering above your client's neck.

Position 6: Place both hands on the upper rib cage, just below the breast line.

> **It is never appropriate to touch any private areas when treating clients.**

Position 7: Place your hands at the Solar Plexus area, above the client's navel.

Position 8: Your hands are now placed one over each pelvic bone.

> **Note: At this point the client is to change positions, from lying on their back to lying on their stomach. Once the client is in position continue treatment.**

Position 9: Place your hands on the client's shoulder blades.

Position 10: Your hands are now placed on the middle back area.

Position 11: Your hand placement is now on the lower back.

Position 12: The final position is the sacral region; place both hand here; and of course follow through with all three steps.

Notes

After completing this part of your Angelic-Reiki Energy Healing Treatment the practitioner should do a complete sweeping of their client's Auric Field, brushing away any debris that may be left over during the client's treatment.

Ask the Client to sit up slowly to get their balance, and then ask them to please sit in a chair for a few minutes.

While the client is getting into a chair, the practitioner should rinse their hands in a basin of lightly salted water; this again neutralizes any left-over energy.

 The practitioner should then offer a bottle of purified water to the client and recommend drinking it. It is also recommended for the Angelic-Reiki practitioner to drink a bottle of purified water at this time. The water will help replenish both their energies.

At this time while you are both sitting and relaxing you may discuss the Client's experience during their Angelic-Reiki Energy Healing Treatment. You should also share your thoughts and messages that you received during their treatment.

<u>Notes</u>

Chapter 5

Different Variations
Of
Angelic-Reiki Healing

Angelic-Reiki: Empowerment Healing Building Confidence through Positive <u>Reinforcement:</u>

Making Changes in Our Thinking

Angelic-Reiki Energy Healing also heals through thoughts and words.

Become Mindful; it will help you to become aware of your thoughts and meditations. Quieting yourself helps in the process of getting in touch with your thoughts. Focusing on Good Health heals and nourishes us. The process of doing the Angelic-Reiki Affirmations' will start to release illness.

Your words are so very powerful, they will change your world; and when adding the Angelic-Reiki Healing Energy to your prayers and affirmations, Miracles are produced.

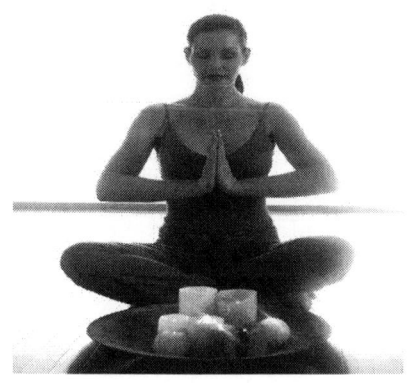

Angelic-Reiki Healing Affirmations will affect your life, creating the reality of harmony and prosperity.

- Speak Happiness and create Joy.

- Speak Well of others and draw the best of people into your life.

- Speak Gratitude and receive Blessing.

- Speak honorably and receive Respect.

- Speak of Good Health and Receive Divine Healing.

- Speak well in all aspects in life and produce the very best in all aspects of your life.

Being mindful of our speech and thoughts will have a wonderful effect on all our relationships and most importantly upon or lives.

An Angelic-Reiki Affirmations can be any positive healing statement, act, or symbolic gesture (such as lighting a candle).

Angelic-Reiki Affirmations

~ For Good Health ~

I am whole and healthy. Every cell in my body is filled with Divine Radiant Healing Angelic-Reiki Energy. I release all sickness and imbalance.

I am now filled with the deep healing energy of the Angelic-Reiki Energy Healing Realm and radiate the very best of health.

Angelic-Reiki Healing Energy flows throughout my body and into the world I give thanks for this Divine Healing.

I give thanks for The Divine Healing Energy of the Angelic-Reiki Angels who rebuild and restores me to perfect health.

I am thankful for my healing.

The Angelic-Reiki Angels heal my body, my emotions, my mind, and my soul.

I am one with the Angelic-Reiki Angels I am healthy, I am healed, and I am Happy.

I choose Happiness knowing with Divine Intervention, Happiness is mine.

The Angelic-Reiki Angels guide me in the choices I make, guiding me with an abundance of healthy choices.

As Angelic-Reiki enters me, my body becomes stronger.

In any and all traditional healing treatment, The Divine Angelic-Reiki Angels activate Divine Healing Energy. I am healed.

I light this Candle activating Angelic-Reiki Healing Energy.

As I place my hand upon my heart the Angelic-Reiki Healing Energy enters my soul healing all past traumas, in all time, in all space in all realms sealed with Divine Healing Grace.

With Angelic-Reiki Energy Healing my body heals quickly and easily.

I am relaxed and filled with Divine Angelic-Reiki Energy, I am filled with peace of mind as my body is repaired, and I heal quickly.

Angelic-Reiki Energy Heals my life.

The Angelic-Reiki Angels assist in my traditional medical treatments.

With every breath I take I inhale Angelic-Reiki Healing Energy.

Angelic-Reiki Energy heals my emotional pain.

Angelic-Reiki Energy nurtures my soul completely filling the emptiness.

I am a Divine Light of Angelic-Reiki Healing Energy and radiate love.

I am grateful.

<u>Notes</u>

<u>Notes</u>

<u>Notes</u>

Angelic-Reiki: Past Lives Healing:

Past-life or Reincarnation is a concept that some people do not believe in, none the less it is true. With this knowledge also comes the knowledge that many of the human beings' fears and illnesses, are carried over from their previous lives.

Past-life traumas that result in these fears and illnesses result from event that happened in the previous lifetime. These traumas are created by significant event that cause us to temporally take us in a different direction on our life path, only for the purpose to teach us a lesson that we would not have learned any other way. Sometime these traumas are too hard for us to heal and learn from so we carry them into the next life-time, this continues until we find a way to heal these traumas and to learn the lessons.

These traumas from past-life may create a host of illnesses, anxieties, fears, unexplained aches and pains. They may also affect our personality, with traits such as low self-esteem, and intimacy issues, and unexplained phobias. These are the shadows that may follow us; through time and space.

Angelic-Reiki Energy Healing helps to heal these past-life traumas, and helps the client to understand the lessons they were to learn, through gentle Angelic-Reiki meditation, this is a slow process, so the healing is complete on all levels, including the DNA cellular level. It is also a slow process preventing any future damage. The client will come away from the Angelic-Reiki Past-Life Healing process a more confident, compassionate, stable, and physically healthy Human Being. They will come away with the knowledge of the lessons they were to have learned so many lifetimes ago. This Angelic-Reiki Past-Life Healing will give clients an opportunity to lead a happier and fulfilled life.

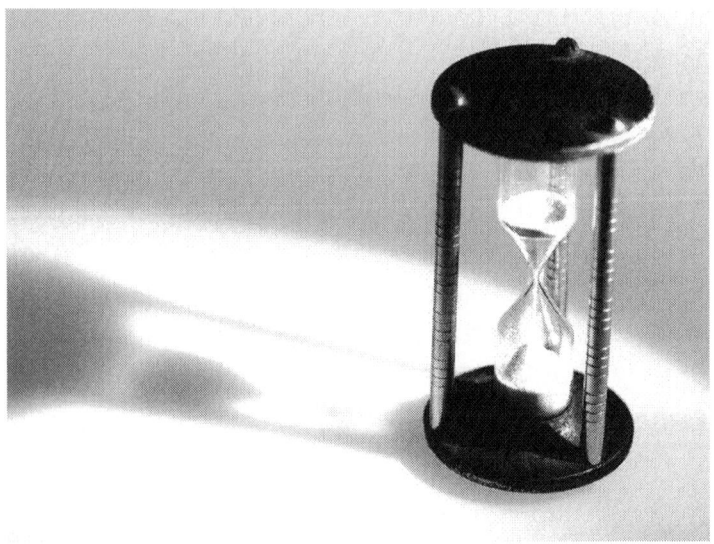

Angelic-Reiki
~Past Life Meditation ~

In the midst of turmoil and pain, when you feel that the very foundation of your world is going to collapse, this is when you should go inward and focus to discover what created this scenario in your life.

Begin asking questions of yourself or your client, these questions,

- Why did I do…

- Who did I hurt…

- Why am I repeating this same scenario…

This is the time for quiet meditation, sit calmly breathing slowly, and with each breath reflect on self-healing. Reflect on inner peace.

Let your thoughts float gentle through your mind, let them float slowly back into time. Regressing you gently back through time, pay attention to your thoughts, to the pictures that appear in your mind.

Deeper and deeper you go into regressions, deep into past life events; discovering powerful and astonishing information about who you are, and why you do what you do.

You are free of all debilitating subconscious fears you feel the Angelic-Reiki Realm of Angels around you, you know you are protected.

You begin to see the events that have plagued you for centuries and the great limitations they had placed on who you are; lifetime after lifetime repeating over and over the same events.

You realize now what you did not know, the knowledge that you could have changed these events; you begin to understand that you now have within you the strength and power to heal these past hurts, these past traumas.

You begin to cry and the emotions that have been blocked for so many lifetimes begin once more to flow. The walls that have kept these emotions in crumble and light begins to enter this lonely empty space. The Light of the Angelic-Reiki Angels begins to fill you.

One by one these past events are encompassed by Divine Healing Angelic-Reiki Light, this healing light penetrates each event, until they burst and no longer exists.

One by one as each event burst into the Divine Healing Light, you feel the heaviness of that burden dissolve; you become lighter.

You begin to breathe deep liberating breaths of fresh air, and with each breath your healing becomes stronger.

Breathing in and out, stronger and stronger you begin to float gently forward it time centuries pass, and with each passing you become lighter.

One deeper breath and you find yourself back in the present. You feel refreshed, renewed, and healed.

You are liberated form these past haunts of time; these false beliefs.

You thank the Angelic-Reiki Angels for their help and protection.

You sit quietly for a few moments in gratitude.

Note: This meditation is a simple exercise. It will remove the past life traumas on the cellular DNA (encoded) level. It is a permanent transformation.

When working with a client this healing meditation should be done at least once a month of a minimum of six months. Each time different events will be healed. This is done slowly to prevent and trauma to the physical being.

Our Sacred Soul is our truth; it rides on the waves of our emotions. Angelic-Reiki Past-Life Healing sets it in motion, to move on an infinite journey of light. Each time we choose our truth and feel our emotions we gain little pieces or our True Sacred Self back from the past; Each time our Divine Light becomes brighter and brighter. We begin to glide through our present life experiences with confidence and grace. We become radiant beings of light, flowing freely for our soul is restored, our soul is complete.

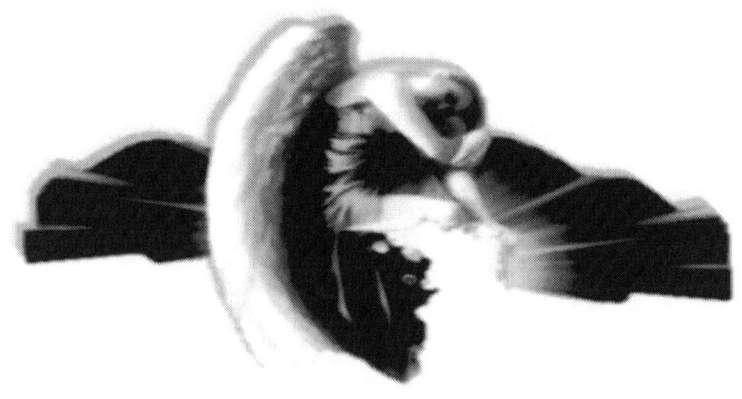

Notes

Notes

Angelic-Reiki
Distance and Situational Healing
(A-RDSH)

Angelic-Reiki Energy Healing for distance and for situational healing **(A-RDSH)** is a technique when the practitioner sends the Angelic-Reiki Healing Angels to bring their healing energies to an absentee client, or a situation that a client is experiencing in their life. I may also be sent through time; so to off-set any ill effects that a client may have before an experience. For example: a Mother may ask for an **A-RDSH**, to be sent for her child before they go for a doctor's visit when a child is going to be receiving an immunization shot. This will lessen any ill effects and the child's experience and it will not so be traumatizing. It may also be sent to a student before they take a test. In this instance the student may not freeze up during the test or go blank, they will also receive clarity of mind. There is no situation that Angelic-Reiki cannot be sent to, and there is no situation that Angelic-Reiki Healing Energy cannot help, this also includes Past-Life Experiences.

Angelic-Reiki Distance Healing encompasses more than this present realm that we currently exist in; it also will travel to the past, healing past-life traumas and it may also be sent to the future, as a preventative. In the same way you may send it to any situation or event in your life or in your client's life.

Begin you're **A-RDSH** by focusing on this truth…

…We are one with God

We are one with the Universe

It is The Divine Truth

That we are

Divinely Entitled

To be

Joyful, Happy,

And

Prosperous

With Divine Intervention

We are blessed

Indeed

Once you have brought your focus to this truth, begin to breath in, feel the Angelic-Reiki Healing Energy entering your Sacred Soul; feel it begin to pulsate throughout your whole body.

Sit quietly for a moment, as the energy builds, begin now to focus on the person or situation you will be sending the Angelic-Reiki Energy Healing to. Place your hands on your lap, palms up; receiving the blessing from the Angelic-Reiki Realm. Feel the connection becoming stronger and stronger.

The practitioner will begin to feel a sense of peacefulness, and warmth as their connection grows. Visualize the Realm of Angelic-Reiki Angels circling around you; with the Angels comes a field of healing energy; this miraculous ball of Healing Angelic-Reiki Light comes to rest in your hands. You begin to focus on the size of the energy ball, it becomes larger and larger; as it grows you begin to focus on the location for the A-RDSH, you begin to see the Angelic-Reiki Energy ball start to float up above your hands, it floats gently up to your Crown Chakra. As it sits above your head this Divine ball of Angelic-Reiki Healing Energy begins to spin, ever faster and faster. Your focus becomes stronger on the healing; the Angelic-Reiki Healing Energy Ball is growing with each turn. Your focus on the A-RDSH is clear, now and you are ready to have the Angels transport the healing.

In a flash the Angelic-Reiki Healing Energy Ball leaves your site; it is now transported through time and through space, to the location of the focused healing.

The practitioner should remain sitting quieting as the A-RDSH is transported to its' healing location. You are now connected to the person or situation and allowing the flow of the Angelic-Reiki Healing Energy to connect to that person or situation. The practitioner should spend as much time as required for the healing; it may be as little as five minutes, or as long as fifteen minutes. It may also help the practitioner to focus by saying the situation or person name that the Angelic-Reiki Energy Healing is being sent to, the practitioner may want to repeat the name of the person or situation several times as the energy is being transported.

Remember when you are finished with the A-RDSH, to express gratitude for the Angelic-Reiki Energy Healing Realm of Angels and The Healing Energy they have shared. You may simply want to light a white candle to express thanks, by all means do this, the Angels love candle light. You will also want to rinse your hands with warm Blessed salted water to ground any excess energy.

A-RDSH Energy Directing Principles

- A-RDSH is always sent for the very best for all concerned, be it for an individual or a situation.

- Understand that the Angelic-Reiki Angelic Realm knows the best way to heal the person or situation. Do not judge the healing.

- It is best to do A-RSDH at a client's request, however if a situation arises (such as an accident) ask for Divine Intervention in reference to sending Angelic-Reiki Healing Energy; and that it will be Divinely Directed and accepted for the person, or situation.

- Not all healing are physical; do not judge the effectiveness of the healing. There is more going on than meets the eye.

> **Note:** **Angelic-Reiki Distance Energy Healing** is an advance form of healing; this type of healing is performed when the client is unable to be present. It is possible to transmit Angelic-Reiki Energy Healing over distance and even through time healing present issues, Past Life issues and Karma. This type of healing is extremely effective. It is a simple way to work with clients even if they are in another state or country.

Notes

Notes

Notes

Chapter 6

Things to Remember:
Angelic-Reiki Procedures

Selecting an Environment:

Just as in Level 1: Any and all Angelic-Reiki Energy Healing Treatments may be done out of the practitioner's home, an office, or an alternative medical clinic; as long as it is a location where both the practitioner and client will be safe and comfortable.

As a practitioner, you may want to set up you own personal Angelic-Reiki Energy Healing Treatment environment to meet your own personal needs. It should be well lit. The location should be a place where you and your client will not be disturbed during *the Angelic-Reiki Energy Healing Session.*

The room should have comfortable chairs and massage table.

A bookcase is also a great idea to have; you may wish to keep blankets, tissues, and note pads for the client to take notes, candles, and music.

Finally, there should be as little distractions as possible

After you have set-up the Healing Room, allow yourself a few moments to relax

<u>Notes</u>

Before You Begin the Angelic-Reiki Treatment:

Prior to appointment ask your client to wear comfortable clothing.

Once your client has arrived, allow the client also to relax after their drive.

Ask your client, what their goals are for the Angelic-Reiki Energy Healing Session.

Ask your client to remove their shoes.

Ask your client if they would rather lie on the table or remain in the chair, explain that lying on the table would be more comfortable.

> **Note: if your client is wheelchair bond, have them remain in the chair for any and all treatments.**

If the client decides to lie on the table put a pillow under the client's knees and head (for their comfort).

Keep tissue and a blanket handy (recipient may experience emotional or physical releases).

Ask your client to keep their legs uncrossed.

Inform your client that Angelic-Reiki will balance and relax the body, and may relieve pain.

Explain that your hands may feel different sensations: such as heat or cold.

Talking during treatment is encouraged; the clients may have insights for you in reference to what they are experiencing, and talking can have a cleansing effect for the client.

Explain to your client that Angelic-Reiki Energy Healing will adjust to the needs and conditions of the client.

During The Angelic-Reiki Treatment:

Let your client know that there are twelve basic hand positions.

You may use a tissue or cloth over face of your client, at their request, during first Head Position.

Do a complete treatment.

Add the additional positions to the client's treatment if you feel directed to do so by the Angelic-Reiki Healing Angels.

Music during treatment will help your client relax.

Use Angelic-Reiki Energy Healing Charge Holy Water™ at the beginning and at the end of each Angelic-Reiki Energy Healing Session.

Notes

After The Angelic-Reiki Treatment:

The practitioner should rinse their hands in a basin of warm water; the water should have one table spoon of **Angelic-Reiki Energy Healing, Blessed Energy Balancing Salts™** dissolved in it, this will ground any excess energy.

Both the practitioner and the client should drink an eight once glass of water at the end of the healing session. This will help restore and balance their energy.

After the client has left the practitioner may want to smudge the Angelic-Reiki Energy Healing Room with white sage. This will clear any energy that may be left in the room.

After the practitioner is done doing Angelic-Reiki Energy Healings for the day, it is advised to take a warm shower and use the Angelic-Reiki Energy Healing Body Wash™. This will help ground and restore the practitioner's energy field.

After showering please allow yourself at least 20 minutes to recoup; you may want to take this time to journal or lay in quiet meditation. You may even fall asleep. (If you fall asleep please pay attention to your dreams, the Angelic-Reiki Angels will bring messages to you.)

Notes

For The Practitioner:

Remember you are Not the healer; The Angelic-Reiki Energy is healing the client. The Angelic-Reiki Energy Healing Angels are working through you.

If the client does not seem to respond immediate to treatment, more treatments may be necessary. The Angelic-Reiki Energy Healing is healing on other levels than just the physical.

In the case of accidents, or emergencies **call 911, we are not medical professionals; and we do not ever treat for any medical condition; unless you are licensed to do so.** After you have call 911 you may send an **A-DSH** to the person or incident.

Never treat a child alone; have a parent present.

Do not diagnose or prescribe anything, unless you are licensed to do so.

Angelic-Reiki works on all levels.

Angelic-Reiki Energy Healing is not just for when a person is sick.

The Angelic-Reiki Energy will add energy to a person, place, thing, situation and relationship.

The Angelic-Reiki Energy Healing may be used on plants, animals, food, etc. Everything will benefit from Angelic-Reiki. It can be used on audio and video tapes, electronic equipment, car batteries, appliances, etc.

Every time you use Angelic- Reiki, you increase the level of Angelic-Reiki Energy brought into this planet, you increase its' love and its' light.

We are all eternal beings through which the Power and Presence of Angelic-Reiki Healing Energy can flow.

The practitioner and the client will be moved from just having faith, to the reality of true belief; and this belief will be comprised of **HOPE**, not of fear.

We as Angelic-Reiki practitioners recognize, and accept, and realty of God and The Angelic Realms; and the perfection of each individual.

We believe that with Divine Intervention All Thing are Possible.

Notes

Notes

Chapter 7

Wrapping Up

Angelic-Reiki Energy Healers are vessels for the Healing Angelic-Reiki Energy to flow through.

Angelic-Reiki Energy Healing

- Promotes natural healing
- Balances the energies in the human body
- Strengthens the immune system
- Treats symptoms and causes of illness
- Relieves pain
- Clears toxins
- Adapts to the needs of the receiver
- Enhances personal awareness
- Relaxes and reduces stress
- Releases blocked and suppressed feelings
- Aids in meditation and positive thinking
- Heals holistically

Remember your recognition of your personal union with the God and The Angelic-Reiki Healing Angels.

Angelic-Reiki Energy Healers is what you have become and how you function and exist now and always.

There can be no compromises, no negotiations with so-called illness or evil.

Those acknowledgements would means denial of good. It is the negative and destructive use of thoughts, feelings, and emotions that must be dissolved.

Take time to observe yourself in all relationship to everyone and everything.

Don't blame others, but look within yourself for causes of outer distress.

Don't fight with the negativity or evil, Realize this Truth; it cannot exist where Light and Love dwells.

By knowing and accepting the Truth, you get rid of mental blocks, such as anger, resentment, grudges, jealousies, etc.

Observe your mood swings and states of thought and feeling.

Practice continued self-examination.

"Know Thy Self"

~ Angelic-Reiki Energy Healing™ ~
**Has but one Principal and in it, is simplicity
That Principal of…**

I Am

I am anger free

I am without worry

I am grateful

I am a diligent worker

I am kind to people

For as I Am

So shall

I Be

My Wish for You

As Always...

May The Powers That Be

Bless You Indeed

With health, wealth

And prosperity

With

Wisdom to share

And

Courage to lead

May They guard your gate

Always keeping safe

Your fate.

Rev. Debbie Michaels

Notes

Notes

Notes

Notes

Notes

Notes

Notes

Notes

<u>Notes</u>

Notes

Notes

Notes

Notes

Notes

Notes

Notes

Notes

Notes

Notes

<u>Notes</u>

Notes

Notes